Natural Care Library

GINSENG

ENERGY ENHANCER

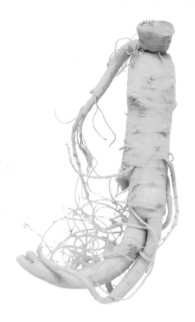

By STEPHANIE PEDERSEN

DORLING KINDERSLEY PUBLISHING, INC.

www.dk.com

CONTENTS

HERBAL HISTORY

Long before over-the-counter medications and prescription drugs came on the scene, herbs proved to be powerful healers. Every culture on earth has used herbal medicine. In fact, herbal usage is older than recorded history itself: Herbal preparations were found in the burial site of a Neanderthal man who lived over 60,000 years ago.

When it comes to herbal medicine, many healing systems are available and useful. Perhaps the best known are ayurveda, Chinese medicine, and Western herbalism. Ayurveda is a system of diagnosis and treatment that uses herbs in conjunction with breathing, meditation, and yoga. It has been practiced in India for more than 2,500 years. Ayurveda gets its name from the Sanskrit words *ayuh*, meaning "longevity," and *veda*, meaning "knowledge." Indeed, in ayurvedic healing, health can be achieved only after identifying a person's physical and mental characteristics (called *dosha*). Then the proper preventative or therapeutic remedies are prescribed to help an individual maintain doshic balance.

Chinese medicine is another healing system that uses herbs, in combination with acupressure, acupuncture, and qi gong. Sometimes called traditional Chinese medicine (TCM), this ancient system is thought to be rooted as far back as 2,800 BC in the time of emperor Sheng Nung. Known as China's patron saint of herbal medicine, Sheng Nung is credited among the first proponents of healing plants. Chinese medicine attempts to help the body correct energy imbalances. Therefore herbs are classified according to certain active characteristics, such as heating, cooling, moisturizing, or drying, and prescribed according to how they influence the activity of various organ systems.

Many herbal practitioners believe that Western herbalism can trace its roots to the ancient Sumerians, who—according to a medicinal recipe dating from 3000 BC—boasted a refined knowledge of herbal medicine. Records from subsequent cultures, such as the Assyrians, Egyptians, Israelites, Greeks, and Romans, show similar herbal healing systems. But these peoples weren't the only ones using beneficial plants. The Celts, Gauls, Scandinavians, and other early European tribes also healed with herbs. In fact, it was their knowledge, melded with the medicine brought by invading Moors and Romans, that formed the foundation for Western herbalism. Simply put, this foundation formed a comprehensive system wherein herbs were grouped according to how they affected both the body and specific body systems.

Western herbalism was refined further when Europeans traveled to the New World. Once here, the Europeans fused their medical knowledge with that of the Native Americans. Herbal know-how became an important part of early American habits, so that wellness remedies were handed down from mothers to daughters to granddaughters, and medicinal plants were grown in home gardens. Physicians from the 1600s, 1700s, 1800s, and early 1900s commonly used plants, such as arnica, echinacea, and garlic to heal patients. Herbs were listed as medicine in official publications such as the *United States Pharmacopoeia* (the definitive American listing) and the *National Formulary* (the pharmacist's handbook). With the creation of synthetic medications in the 1930s, herbal medicine began to wane.

Fortunately, Europeans and Asians never gave up their herbal remedies. Instead, they used them to complement synthetic medications. Their successes—combined with the desire of many Americans for alternatives to the high price tags and unforgiving side effects of synthetic drugs—have kept the world moving forward on a healthier herbal path.

What Is Ginseng?

Ginseng is among today's most popular herbal remedies. Walk the aisles of any health store and you can't miss it: ginseng in capsules, liquid extracts, teas, tinctures, and more. Yet ginseng is no medicinal newcomer—the herb boasts a long, distinguished history as an adaptogen, tonic, central nervous system stimulant and circulatory stimulant. Centuries of Chinese healers have used it to fight such wide-ranging ills as low blood pressure, general weakness, malaise, mental deficiency and sexual dysfunction. In fact, some of the earliest recorded usages of the herb—to increase libido and strengthen "weak mentality"—come from Emperor Shen Nung, who began his reign in 2800 BC and is considered China's patron saint of herbal medicine. He wrote the Chinese herbal tome *The Herbal Classic of the Divine Plowman*.

At one time ginseng grew wild throughout China and Korea. Today, Chinese ginseng is extremely rare in the wild, but it is cultivated in the US, China, Korea and Russia. A member of the Araliaceae family, ginseng is a low-growing perennial that is difficult to cultivate. The plant's medicinal portion is the root—yet the root doesn't become ready for harvesting until the plant's sixth, seventh, or eighth autumn.

Today, ginseng is best known as a revitalizer and a stimulant that is especially helpful in boosting immune-system function, increasing red blood cell count, and combating fatigue, general weakness, loss of mental acuity and edema—all of which may occur among those who are in a state of stress or poor health. Among the herb's compounds are a group of 13 different triterpenoid saponins known collectively as ginsenosides. Other compounds include B-complex vitamins, choline, flavonoids, panacene (a volatile oil), pectin, sterols, polyacetylene derivatives, and polysaccharides.

Yet there's more to ginseng than its "stimulating" qualities. The herb has long been used to combat high blood sugar in diabetics provide protection against radiation (as well as treat radiation damage) and enhance the body's antibody responses to marauding infections. Currently, test-tube studies indicate that ginseng has anticancer qualities.

IN OTHER WORDS
Like many herbs, Ginseng is known by several names. Here are a few of them:

✦ Asian Ginseng
✦ Chinese Ginseng
✦ Jeng Seng
✦ Korean Ginseng
✦ Man Root
✦ Panax Ginseng
✦ Ren Shen
✦ Shin Seng

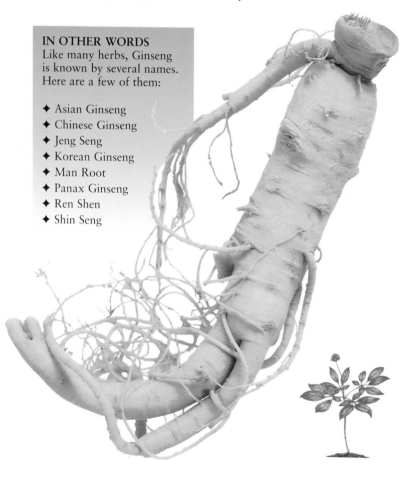

SCIENCE TALK

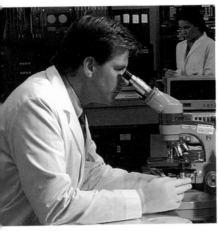

MEDICINE WORLDWIDE
The National Institutes of Health, in Bethesda, MD, estimate that only 10 to 30 percent of the health care worldwide is allopathic, or "Western." The rest of the world's medical care is what Americans would call "alternative," including ayurveda, energy healing, herbalism, homeopathy and traditional Chinese medicine.

CELEBRATING GERMAN KNOW-HOW
Perhaps no other country in the Western world has done more than Germany to further the cause of herbal medicine. What's the country's secret? Commission E, a review board of respected pharmacologists, physicians and scientists. The board was established in 1978, and members spent the first 15 years researching more than 300 age-old herbal remedies for usages, recommended dosages, preparations and side effects. Then, in 1980, the German government upped the medical ante, creating a mandate requiring all new herbal remedies sold in pharmacies to meet the same criteria as over-the-counter drugs. To comply, researchers performed thousands of rigorous clinical trials, resulting in a deep well of knowledge used by doctors open to herbs worldwide.

DO YOU HAVE A CONTRAINDICATION?

Before taking any herb, it's important to ask your physician whether you have any contraindications. What does contraindication mean? It's a common medical term that refers to a symptom or condition that makes a particular treatment inadvisable. For example, when it comes to ginseng, high blood pressure is a contraindication. Why? Adding the stimulating powers of ginseng to this mix can create an even greater health hazard.

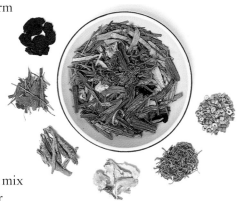

Before taking any herb, ask yourself the following questions:

✔ Have I done any background research on the herb?

✔ What condition am I taking this herb for?

✔ Am I taking other medications or herbs that may affect the herb's functioning?

✔ Do I have any pre-existing condition that is contraindicated?

✔ Am I pregnant, trying to conceive or nursing?

✔ Have I spoken to my physician, a naturopathic doctor or an herbalist before taking herb?

✔ Do I know the proper dosages for the herb?

RETHINKING MEDICATION

ANTIBIOTICS: ARE THEY ESSENTIAL?

A recent report published in the *Journal of the American Medical Association* stated that even though antibiotics provide little help for colds, upper respiratory tract infections and bronchitis, doctors still prescribe antibiotics for these conditions. Why? In part, because patients expect their doctors to give them some kind of medication, and many physicians find it easier to oblige than take time out to explain how antibiotics do and don't work. Americans are so enamored of antibiotics that doctors write over 12 million antibiotic prescriptions annually. To learn more about the dangers of antibiotic abuse, contact the Centers For Disease Control and Prevention, 404-332-4555.

PENICILLIN BY THE POUND

Since penicillin's debut in 1941, antibiotic production has shot up from 2 million pounds in 1954 to more than 50 million pounds in 1997. Where is all this medication going? Half of the antibiotics produced annually are prescribed for people; the rest are mixed into livestock feed and used as fertilizers for agricultural crops. The downside to this free-flowing penicillin? New, strong, antibiotic-resistant strains of bacteria.

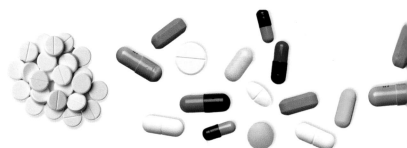

WAIT! BEFORE YOU TAKE THAT PILL . . .
Before asking your doctor for an antibiotic, ask yourself the following questions:

✔ Is my condition caused by bacteria? If not, antibiotics will not work.

✔ Are antibiotics necessary for recovery? If the infection will go away on its own, consider forgoing antibiotics.

✔ Are there alternatives to antibiotics? If herbal or other natural remedies can fight off the infection, consider using one or more of them.

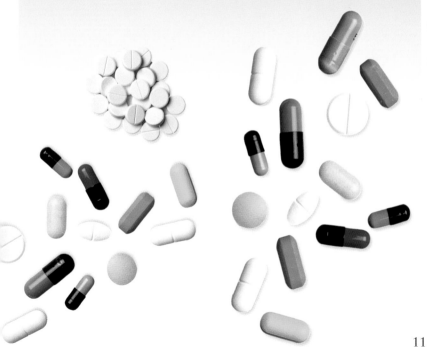

COMMON SIDE EFFECTS

Like many medicinal herbs, ginseng can cause mild side effects. Here's what a small number of users experience:

+ Diarrhea
+ Headache
+ Heart palpitations
+ Heavier menstrual flow
+ Irritability
+ Insomnia
+ Restlessness

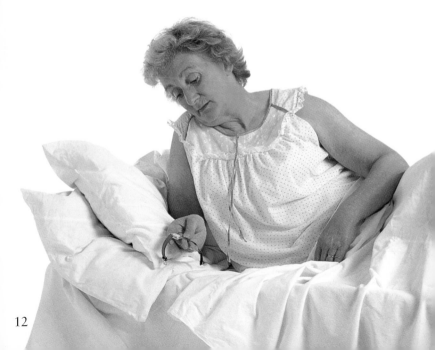

PRECAUTIONS

✖ The doses in this book are generally aimed at adults. We strongly suggest consulting your child's physician before administering ginseng externally or internally. If your physician does okay ginseng for your child, we generally recommend halving the adult doses suggested in this book. Again, please consult your child's physician.

✖ Do not self-medicate with ginseng while taking any type of anticoagulant medication. To do so can thin the blood too much, leading to possible internal bleeding. For information on how to safely switch from a synthetic anticoagulant to ginseng, talk to your physician.

✖ Do not self-medicate with ginseng while taking any type of vasodilator medication. To do so can overdilate blood vessels. For information on how to safely switch from a synthetic anticoagulant to ginseng, talk to your physician.

✖ If you are pregnant, nursing, trying to conceive or are taking any type of medication, please consult your physician before using ginseng.

✖ To avoid dangerous interactions between prescription medication and herbal medicine, individuals with AIDS, cancer, a connective tissue disease, heart disease, kidney disease, liver disease, tuberculosis, or any other chronic illness should consult their physician before using any herb.

FORMULA GUIDE

Capsules, extracts, teas, tinctures—what do they all mean?
For the uninitiated, we offer this guide to herbal formulas:

✦ **Capsules.** The medicinal part of the herb is freeze dried, pulverized and packed into gelatin capsules. Capsules usually contain 200 mg of herb powder; occasionally the dried herb is reinforced with concentrated extracts.

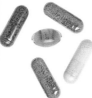

✦ **Herb, Dried.** The flowers, leaves, stems and/or roots of many herbs are often available dried at health food stores and Chinese pharmacies. While these are most commonly made into homemade teas, they can also be used to make decoctions, infused oils, sachets and more.

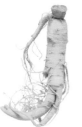

✦ **Herb, Fresh.** Herbs that are used in both culinary and medicinal ways (such as parsley or dill) are most often found fresh. These can be made into homemade extract, juice, infused oil, teas and more.

✦ **Juices.** The extracted juice from fresh herbs can be found mixed with commercially prepared fruit or vegetable juices.

✦ **Liquid Extract** (also called Extract). Macerated plant material is percolated in a solvent such as glycerin or water and used undiluted. Generally stronger than a tincture.

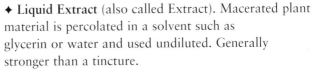

✦ **Oil, Essential** (also called Oil). Essential oils are the volatile oily components of herbs. They are found in tiny glands located in the flowers, leaves, roots and/or bark and are mechanically or chemically extracted. Essential oil is used externally.

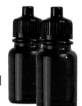

✦ **Oil, Infused.** Made by steeping fresh or dried herbs in an edible oil. After a period of time, the herbs are removed and the oil is used internally or externally. Not as potent as essential oil.

✦ **Ointments.** Dried or fresh herbs are steeped in a base of oils and emulsifiers (such as beeswax, petroleum jelly or soft paraffin wax). After a period of time, the herbs are removed and the ointment packaged. For external use only.

✦ **Syrups.** Syrups are generally a combination of herbal extracts and a sweetener, such as honey or sugar. Generally used for colds, flu and sore throats.

✦ **Teas/Infusions.** The words "tea" and "infusion" are often used interchangeably in herbal medicine. While commercial herbal tea bags are available, herbal tea can also be made with loose dried or fresh herbs.

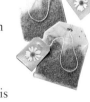

✦ **Tinctures.** Plant material is soaked in alcohol. The saturated plant material is then pressed. Liquid from this pressing is diluted with water and packaged—usually in small dropper bottles.

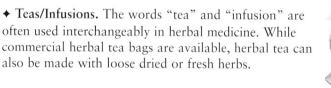

CONDITIONS AND DOSES

FATIGUE

❒ **Symptoms:** Fatigue is a side effect of many medical and nonmedical conditions, including depression, illness, mental exertion, physical exertion, and stress. Signs of fatigue include mental and physical exhaustion, lethargy, sleepiness and general weakness.

❒ **How Ginseng Can Help:** In Chinese medicine, ginseng is the herb of choice to combat fatigue—regardless of the underlying cause. Both animal and human studies have found ginseng's tonic effects stimulate the central nervous system, improve energy metabolism during exercise, boost metabolic activity in the brain, and stimulate nerve impulses in muscles— all of which can improve mental and physical performance.

❒ **Dosages:** During periodic times of fatigue, enjoy 1 to 3 cups a day of ginseng tea. Ginseng can also be used as a daily supplement to help combat long-term fatigue—however, before taking ginseng, speak with your physician about whether the herb is for you. The dosage is one 200-mg capsule twice a day; or 1/2 teaspoon of liquid extract twice a day; or 1 teaspoon of tincture twice a day. If taking ginseng for an extended period, plan on taking a one-week break from the herb every four or five weeks. This reduces the chance of possible hypertension, insomnia or restlessness that some health authorities believe can develop with long-term ginseng usage.

NIGHT-DUTY AID

Ginseng has long been celebrated for its energizing properties. To test these powers, a British researcher named Stephen Fulder studied a group of nurses who had switched from day shifts to night shifts. After rating themselves for competence, fatigue, mood and well-being, the nurses were given mental and physical performance tests. The group was then split in two, half given ginseng, the other half given a placebo. The result? At the end of their work shifts, the nurses who took ginseng rated their moods as higher and their fatigue as less. They also scored better on speed and coordination tests.

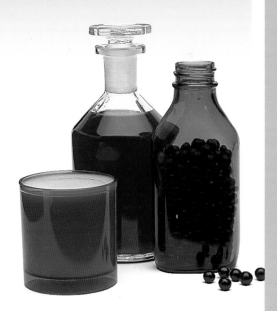

CONDITIONS AND DOSES

STRESS

❐ **Symptoms:** Who doesn't experience periods of stress? Whether caused by increased demands at work, money worries, relationship woes, or something else entirely, stress can cause changes in appetite, gastrointestinal upset, headaches, impaired concentration, irritability, muscle tension, sleeplessness, and teeth-grinding.

❐ **How Ginseng Can Help:** Several American and European studies have found that ginseng enhances the body's ability to cope with stress. First, ginseng controls the release of adrenocorticotropic hormone, an adrenal steroid that increases in response to stress. Very simply put, the less of this steroid in the body, the weaker the body's physical response to stress. Secondly, ginseng maintains steady levels of ascorbic acid in the adrenal gland. This is important because when the body is stressed, levels of ascorbic acid in the adrenal gland plummet. Both these actions help the body maintain a sense of physical calm.

❐ **Dosages:** During periodic stressful times, enjoy 1 to 3 cups a day of ginseng tea. Ginseng can also be used as a daily supplement to help combat long-term stress—however, before taking ginseng, speak with your physician about whether the herb is for you. The dosage is one 200-mg capsule twice a day; or 1/2 teaspoon of liquid extract twice a day; or 1 teaspoon of tincture twice a day. If taking ginseng for an extended period, plan on taking a one-week break from the herb every four or five weeks. This reduces the chance of possible hypertension, insomnia or restlessness that some health authorities believe can develop with long-term ginseng usage.

GINSENG ABUSE SYNDROME

Because ginseng is known as an all-around tonic, many people take it for literally whatever ails them. Unfortunately, indiscriminate ginseng use can cause problems. In the medical world there is a condition known as ginseng abuse syndrome, or GAS. Like its name states, the syndrome is caused by ginseng abuse. This abuse can occur when individuals who do not need ginseng take it, when the dose ingested is too high, or when ginseng is taken regularly over too long a period.

Symptoms include feelings of euphoria, hypertension, insomnia, morning diarrhea, nervousness, rashes and/or shortness of breath. Because each individual's response to any herb is unique, it is important to be alert for potential signs of ginseng abuse.

CONDITIONS AND DOSES

SUSCEPTIBILITY TO INFECTIOUS ILLNESSES

❏ **Symptoms:** The average American gets two or three colds and one bout of flu each year. If you suffer from more than this, there's a chance you may have a poorly functioning immune system—which increases your susceptibility to infectious illnesses. Some people are born with weak immune systems, while others undermine their immunity with heavy drinking, poor diet, recreational drug use, smoking, or chronic stress.

❏ **How Ginseng Can Help:** Ginseng boasts immunity-boosting powers. American studies have found that it enhances the activity of macrophages, white blood cells that detoxify the blood and lymphatic system by destroying bacteria, viruses, and other waste matter. This, in turn, increases the body's defense system.

❏ **Dosages:** During cold and flu season, enjoy 1 to 3 cups a day of ginseng tea. Or, take one 200-mg capsule twice a day; or 1/2 teaspoon of liquid extract twice a day; or 1 teaspoon of tincture twice a day. If taking ginseng for an extended period, plan on taking a one-week break from the herb every four or five weeks. This reduces the chance of possible hypertension, insomnia or restlessness that some health authorities believe can develop with long-term ginseng usage.

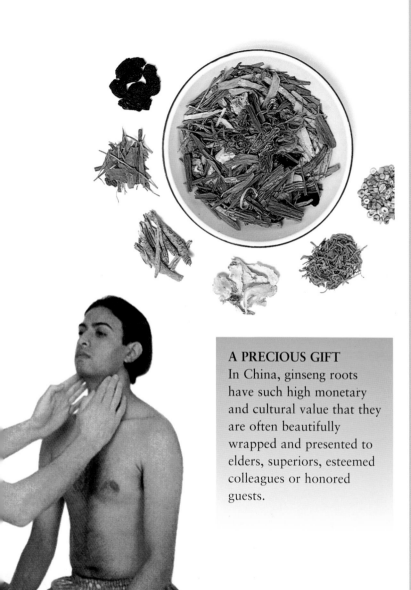

A PRECIOUS GIFT
In China, ginseng roots have such high monetary and cultural value that they are often beautifully wrapped and presented to elders, superiors, esteemed colleagues or honored guests.

CONDITIONS AND DOSES

CANCER

❒ **Symptoms:** Cancer occurs when cells begin growing abnormally, forming malignant tumors. These malignant tumors can appear in the breast, the bones, the throat, the brain, the stomach—actually, in almost any area of the body. But why do cells begin acting strangely in the first place? It's believed that exposure to carcinogens can cause body cells to mutate. Common carcinogens include cigarette smoke, fatty foods, industrial chemicals, insecticides, nuclear radiation, pesticides used on food, polluted air, and ultraviolet light. While cancer symptoms vary widely depending on what part of the body is affected, general signs include blood in the urine or stool, fatigue, hoarseness, indigestion, nagging cough, sores that do not heal, thickening somewhere in the body, and unexplained weight loss.

❒ **How Ginseng Can Help:** In a large international study, individuals who took ginseng on a daily basis had significantly lower cancer rates than individuals who didn't take ginseng. It works by neutralizing various chemical carcinogens, including urethane and aflatoxin. The herb not only protects against cancer, but as shown in clinical studies, shrinks existing tumors.

❒ **Dosages:** As a preventative, take one 200-mg capsule twice a day; or 1/2 teaspoon of liquid extract twice a day; or 1 teaspoon of tincture twice a day. With your physician's recommendation, the same dosage can be taken as a complementary therapy to radiation and/or chemotherapy. If taking ginseng continually, plan on taking a one-week break from the herb every four or five weeks. This reduces the chance of possible hypertension, insomnia or restlessness that some health authorities believe can develop with long-term ginseng usage.

RADIATION SHIELD

Radiation is everywhere. It's in sunlight, microwave ovens, X rays, and radon gas in the home. The average American is exposed to approximately 360 mrad of ionizing radiation each year. X rays alone account for 11 percent of most people's yearly exposure to radiation. An mrad is a small unit of radiation measurement; ionizing radiation refers to the type of radiation which penetrates the body. True, much of this radiation is unavoidable—but it can still lead to cancer. Fortunately, there may be a way to defend yourself. In two separate studies, daily intake of ginseng was shown to protect against radiation damage. When using ginseng as a protectant, take one 200-mg capsule twice a day; or 1/2 teaspoon of liquid extract, twice a day; or 1 teaspoon of tincture twice a day. If taking ginseng for an extended period, plan on taking a one-week break from the herb every four or five weeks. This reduces the chance of possible hypertension, insomnia or restlessness that some health authorities believe can develop with long-term ginseng usage.

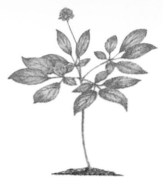

CONDITIONS AND DOSES

ANEMIA

❐ **Symptoms:** Anemia, also called iron-deficiency anemia, occurs when there is not enough iron in the body. Without the proper amount of this mineral, the body cannot produce adequate amounts of hemoglobin. Why does this matter? Hemoglobin is responsible for carrying tissue-nourishing oxygen from the lungs to every part of the body. Without oxygen, the body cannot function properly. A low-iron diet, heavy monthly menstrual flow, pregnancy, lead poisoning, recent blood loss or poor iron absorption by the body can all lead to anemia. Initial signs are so mild they often pass unnoticed: fatigue that is greater than usual, or slight pallor. Later on, the heart rate may grow faster, and the sufferer become winded more easily than usual.

❐ **How Ginseng Can Help:** Doctors of Chinese medicine have longed used ginseng to counteract anemia. In this country, however, iron supplements are the most common treatment for anemia. Fortunately, the two therapies complement each other: The ginsenosides in ginseng have been found by several Japanese and Chinese studies to increase iron uptake in the blood, thus helping the body better absorb iron from supplements.

❐ **Dosages:** Take one 200-mg capsule twice a day; or 1/2 teaspoon of liquid extract twice a day; or 1 teaspoon of tincture twice a day.

HIGH BLOOD CHOLESTEROL

❏ **Symptoms:** High blood cholesterol refers to high levels of fat in the blood. Blame the condition on a fatty diet, heredity, alcoholism, smoking, sedentary lifestyle, or a combination thereof—whatever the cause, the condition is dangerous. Gummy in texture, fat thickens blood and gets stuck on artery walls, thus increasing one's risk of coronary artery disease, heart attack, and stroke. Symptoms can include chest pain, lethargy, pallor and shortness of breath. However, the condition is often asymptomatic; many individuals learn they have high cholesterol only after a routine blood test.

❏ **How Ginseng Can Help:** Taking ginseng is one of many complementary measures that lower high blood cholesterol levels. Important steps include adopting a low-fat vegetarian or near-vegetarian diet, quitting smoking, and exercising regularly. Several American, Chinese and Japanese studies have found that ginseng works with more traditional therapies by reducing total levels of serum cholesterol, triglycerides, and fatty acids and thinning fat-thickened blood. Ginseng also accelerates the body's excretion of cholesterol.

❏ **Dosages:** If you are currently on medication to lower blood cholesterol level, talk to your doctor about replacing medication with ginseng. Take one 200-mg capsule twice a day; or 1/2 teaspoon of liquid extract twice a day; or 1 teaspoon of tincture twice a day.

CONDITIONS AND DOSES

HYPOTENSION

❒ **Symptoms:** Blood pressure refers to the amount of blood pumped by the heart into the arteries. Most people have heard of hypertension, or high blood pressure. But low blood pressure, while not as dangerous as the high type, can also be hazardous. Called hypotension, low blood pressure is caused by diabetes, heredity, illness, medications, or pregnancy. The condition makes it difficult for fresh, oxygen-rich blood to travel through the body. Thus, people with hypotension report cold hands and feet, and tingling limbs, faintness upon standing as well as symptoms caused by lack of blood to the extremities and head, respectively.

❒ **How Ginseng Can Help:** Individuals with hypotension are often advised to use caution upon rising and to change positions carefully. Ginseng can also help. Doctors of Chinese medicine have traditionally used ginseng to strengthen a weak or sluggish heart muscle and American studies have shown that the herb both elevates blood pressure and improves blood supply to the brain.

❒ **Dosages:** Take one 200-mg capsule twice a day; or 1/2 teaspoon of liquid extract twice a day; or 1 teaspoon of tincture twice a day.

TYPES OF GINSENG

There are many species of ginseng: American ginseng, Japanese ginseng, Siberian ginseng, tienchi ginseng, and more—each variety containing different medicinal compounds and healing properties and used to treat different illnesses. Yet this book focuses on panax ginseng, also known as Asian, Chinese or Korean ginseng. Why? First, this particular variety appears to be the most powerful of the ginseng family. Second, Chinese, American and European research and usage has concentrated solely on panax ginseng—making its benefits the most thoroughly documented of the ginseng family.

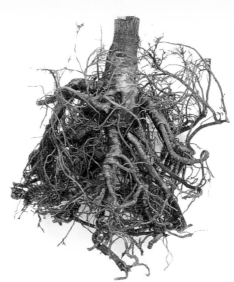

Siberian Ginseng

CONDITIONS AND DOSES

DIABETES

❐ **Symptoms:** To understand diabetes, it helps to know something about the pancreas. The organ—long and thin and situated behind the stomach—is responsible for regulating the body's use of glucose. To do so, the pancreas creates a number of chemicals, including insulin. When blood glucose levels begin to rise, it is insulin's job to prod muscle and fat cells to absorb whatever glucose they need for future activities; the liver stores any surplus. Yet some individuals either do not produce enough insulin (Type 1 diabetes), or their body resists whatever insulin is produced (Type 2 diabetes), thus making an outside source necessary. Either way, the result is the same. Type 1, or juvenile-onset diabetes, typically affects children and young adults and is genetically-linked. Type 2, or adult-onset diabetes, occurs in adults and is linked to obesity. Symptoms of both types include blurred vision, fatigue, frequent bladder infections, increased appetite, increased thirst, increased urination, nausea, skin infections, vaginitis, and vomiting. If not treated, diabetes type 1 and type 2 can cause blood vessel damage, gangrene, heart attack, kidney damage, nerve damage, stroke and vision problems.

❐ **How Ginseng Can Help:** Ginseng is a popular diabetes treatment that can be used alone or in tandem with traditional medication. The herb's adenosine and polysaccharides lower above normal blood sugar levels. Furthermore, ginseng has been shown to promote insulin secretion in diabetics—even though the herb does not have this affect on nondiabetics.

❏ **Dosages:** Before taking ginseng, speak with your physician about whether the herb is for you. This is especially important if you are currently on medication for diabetes. The recommended dose is one 200-mg capsule twice a day; or 1/2 teaspoon of liquid extract twice a day; or 1 teaspoon of tincture twice a day. If taking ginseng continually, plan on taking a one-week break from the herb every four or five weeks. This reduces the chance of possible hypertension, insomnia or restlessness that some health authorities believe can develop with long-term ginseng usage.

RAISE THE DEAD
Chinese medicine often uses large amounts of ginseng to temporarily revive individuals whose death is near. In ancient China, when it became apparent that a ruler was about to die, enormous amounts of ginseng were administered—sometimes up to an entire root a day. This revived the individual for a few extra hours or days, giving him or her a chance to summon loved ones, get affairs in order, and say good-byes before passing on. This practice continues today.

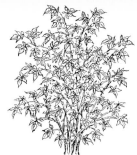

CONDITIONS AND DOSES

IMPOTENCE

❏ **Symptoms:** While anything from too much alcohol to anger to depression can cause short-term erectile problems, impotence is defined as a chronic inability to have or sustain an erection. It is believed that as many as 30 million American men suffer from the condition. In 90 percent of the cases, an organic cause is the culprit—usually diminished blood flow caused by fatty deposits in the arteries leading from the heart to the penis.

❏ **How Ginseng Can Help:** In Chinese medicine, ginseng is regularly prescribed to treat impotence. Indeed, in animal studies, ginseng has been shown to increase testosterone levels and sperm count, both of which can promote more sustained erections.

❏ **Dosages:** Take one 200-mg capsule twice a day; or 1/2 teaspoon of liquid extract twice a day; or 1 teaspoon of tincture twice a day. If taking ginseng continually, plan on taking a one-week break from the herb every four or five weeks. This reduces the chance of possible hypertension, insomnia or restlessness that some health authorities believe can develop with long-term ginseng usage.

LOW LIBIDO

❏ **Symptoms:** *Libido* is a Latin word meaning "sexual drive." Today, if someone talks of a low libido, he or she is referring to a low desire for sex. Of course, there are many reasons one doesn't feel like having sex, including anger toward a partner, bad body image, fatigue, low self-esteem, negative attitude toward sex, physical illness and more. Sometimes, however, there is no concrete reason.

❏ **How Ginseng Can Help:** Ginseng has long been touted as a sexual rejuvenator and is prescribed by doctors of Chinese medicine to increase libido. Although human studies have not been performed proving this, several animal studies have shown that ginseng increases sexual activity and mating behavior in rats. That said, however, it is important to examine any possible underlying causes of low libido—such as anger or low self-esteem—before trying ginseng.

❏ **Dosages:** If there is no explainable reason for low libido, take one 200-mg capsule twice a day; or 1/2 teaspoon of liquid extract twice a day; or 1 teaspoon of tincture, twice a day. Discontinue once your sexual appetite returns.

CONDITIONS AND DOSES

MENOPAUSE

❒ **Symptoms:** Menopause is not an illness but a natural condition that occurs when the ovaries no longer produce enough estrogen to stimulate the lining of the uterus and vagina. Simply put, menopause is when women no longer menstruate or get pregnant. It generally occurs somewhere between the ages of 40 and 60. One of the most famous signs of menopause is the hot flash, a sudden reddening of the face accompanied by a feeling of intense warmth. Other common symptoms include depressed mood, fluid retention, insomnia, irritability, nervousness, night sweats, painful intercourse, rapid heart beat, susceptibility to bladder problems, thinning of vaginal tissues, vaginal dryness, and weight gain. It should be noted that some women experience few symptoms, while still others encounter none at all.

❒ **How Ginseng Can Help:** One traditional remedy for menopause is hormone replacement therapy. This optional treatment uses synthetic hormones to elevate progesterone and estrogen to their premenopausal levels. Ginseng is helpful regardless of whether one undergoes or forgoes hormone replacement therapy. Ginsenosides have an estrogen-like action on vaginal walls. This helps prevent the tissue thinning and painful dryness that many menopausal women experience.

❑ **Dosages:** Take one 200-mg capsule three times a day; or 1/2 teaspoon of liquid extract three times a day; or 1 teaspoon of tincture three times a day. With your physician's recommendation, the same dosage can be taken as a complementary treatment to hormone replacement therapy. If taking ginseng continually, plan on taking a one-week break from the herb every four or five weeks. This reduces the chance of possible hypertension, insomnia or restlessness that some health authorities believe can develop with long-term ginseng usage.

ELDER CARE
Throughout Asia, ginseng is used most often by individuals over 40 for weakness, low energy, and to recover after fever or illness. Ginseng is also used as a general tonic for older people—even those in good health—especially in the winter months. As expensive as ginseng is in developing Asian countries, families try to keep enough of the costly herb on hand to treat any health crisis their respected elders might suffer.

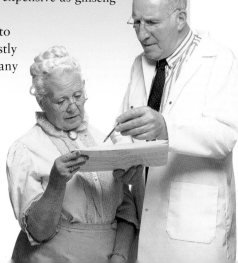

DO-IT-YOURSELF REMEDIES

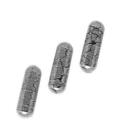

✦ **Capsule:** Make your own herb supplements by purchasing animal or vegetable gelatin capsules at your local health food store and packing each individual capsule with 200 mg of dried, powdered ginseng root.

✦ **Decoction:** Because ginseng root is less permeable than the aerial parts of the plant, simmering the root in boiling water helps extract a greater percentage of its medicinal constituents. To make a decoction, place 25 grams of chopped dried root or 75 grams of chopped fresh root in a nonreactive saucepan. Cover with 750 ml of cold water, place a lid on the saucepan, and boil until the liquid reduces to 500 ml—this usually takes from 20 to 40 minutes. Strain the liquid. Use warm or allow to cool.

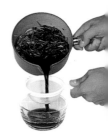

✦ **Drying:** Wash, thoroughly dry and chop fresh ginseng into small pieces. Lay the chopped root on trays in a dry, well-ventilated, nonsunny area of your home or place in an extremely low oven, making sure air is continually circulating around the herbs. Or you can use a dehydrator. Drying will take between two and five days. When drying herbs either in a warm room or an oven, the temperature should be kept between 70° to 90° F. Store dried root in a dark, airtight container.

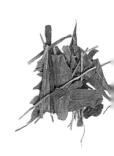

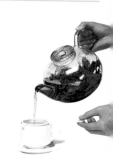

◆ **Fomentation:** Fomentations are essentially gauze or surgical bandages that are soaked in freshly made herbal tea. The hot cloth is then laid directly on a bite, rash or wound.

◆ **Infused Oil Made With Fresh or Dried Root:**
To make ginseng oil, place 200 g of dried ginseng root in a nonreactive saucepan and cover with 500 ml of almond or olive oil. Simmer over very low heat for three hours. Allow mixture to cool. Strain the oil and store it in a dark, airtight container for up to two years. Can be ingested or used externally.

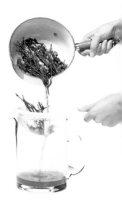

◆ **Liquid Extract.** Also known as extract. To make ginseng extract, macerate 100 to 200 g of dried ginseng root, or 300 to 500 g of fresh ginseng root. Place the herb in a jar and pour in 335 ml vodka (37 proof or higher) and 165 ml water. Place the lid on the jar and store in a dark area for four to eight weeks. Shake the mixture daily. When ready, strain the mixture, pressing all remaining liquid from the ginseng. Place liquid in a nonreactive saucepan and simmer over medium heat for 20 to 40 minutes until the liquid has been reduced by a third. This process burns off the alcohol, leaving the medicinal liquid behind. Allow liquid to cool and decant into several dropper bottles or a clean glass bottle. Will keep up to two years. Shake before using.

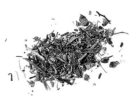

Do-It-Yourself Remedies

✦ Ointment: Also called a salve, herbal ointment is easy to make at home. To create your own ginseng ointment, mix 1 to 2 parts beeswax or soft paraffin wax, 7 parts cocoa butter, and 3 parts powdered ginseng in a nonreactive saucepan. Cook the mixture for one to two hours on a low setting. Let cool, package in an airtight container, and apply up to three times a day.

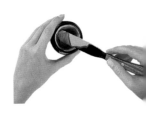

✦ Poultice: Fresh herbs can be applied directly to the skin when fashioned into a poultice. To make a ginseng poultice, chop fresh or dried root. Boil in a small amount of water for five minutes (or use a microwave). Squeeze out any excess liquid from the boiled herb (reserve liquid). Lay the ginseng directly on the skin and cover with a warm moist towel. Leave in place for up to 30 minutes. The reserved liquid can be rewarmed and used to reheat the towel.

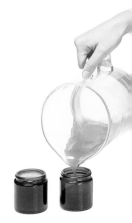

✦ Syrup: Ginseng's taste may not be palatable to some individuals. Syrup delivers the herb's medicinal benefits in an easy-to-swallow (and throat-soothing) base. To make, mix 7 parts ginseng tea or decoction in a nonreactive saucepan with 10 parts sugar. Cook the mixture over low heat until it has formed a thick, syrupy consistency.

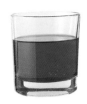

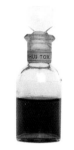

◆ **Tea:** Also known as an infusion, tea is an easy and common way to ingest an herb. To make ginseng tea, steep 1 teaspoon dried root or 1 tablespoon fresh leaves for five minutes in 1 cup of boiling water. You may add fructose, sugar or honey to sweeten.

◆ **Tinctures:** Though they are not as potent as liquid extracts, tinctures are minimally processed, making them a favorite remedy of many herbalists. To make your own ginseng tincture, place 100 to 200 g of dried ginseng, or 300 to 500 g of fresh ginseng, in a large jar and cover with 500 ml vodka (37 proof or higher). Place the lid on the jar and store in a dark area for four to six weeks. Shake the bottle daily. When ready to use, strain the mixture, pressing all remaining liquid from the ginseng. Decant into several dropper bottles or a clean glass bottle. Will keep for up to two years. Shake before using.

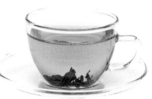

ALTERNATIVE HEALTH STRATEGIES

Herbs, vitamins, minerals—sure these contribute to good health.
But creating general well-being involves more than simply taking
supplements. Good health has to do with various quality of life
issues that can aggravate or cause stress, thus harming health.
Here are some additional ways to help keep yourself well.

Improve Your Eating Habits

Here are the five main eating strategies people follow; consider
finding the healthiest one that works with your lifestyle.

- OMNIVORE
- PISCATORIAL
- MACROBIOTIC
- VEGAN
- VEGETARIAN

Get More Exercise

Whether it's walking or weightlifting, any type of exercise can help
you feel better. Try any of these types:

- STRETCHING
- AEROBICS
- STRENGTH TRAINING

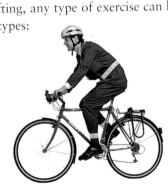

Simple Ways To Ease Stress

In addition to exercise and healthy eating, here are some more techniques–old and new–for easing stress and increasing relaxation.

- GET ENOUGH SLEEP
- MEDITATE REGULARLY
- GIVE UP JUNK FOOD
- ADOPT A PET
- SURROUND YOURSELF WITH SUPPORTIVE PEOPLE
- LIMIT YOUR EXPOSURE TO CHEMICALS
- TAKE YOUR VITAMINS
- ENJOY YOURSELF

ONE-MINUTE STRESS REDUCER

Stress is one of the top health hazards we face today. Unfortunately, it's impossible to go through life without the irritations that make us tense. Fortunately, there *is* something you can do to minimize their power to aggravate you. It's called deep breathing, and it can be done anywhere and anytime you need to calm and center yourself. Here's how it works:

1. Inhale deeply through your nose.
2. Hold your breath for up to three seconds, then exhale your breath through your mouth.
3. Continue as needed.

Deep breathing pulls a person's attention away from a given stressor and refocuses it on his or her breath. This type of breathing is not only comforting (thanks to its rhythmic quality), but also has been shown to lower rapid pulse and shallow respiration—two temporary symptoms of stress.

GET MOVING

Ask medical experts to name one stay-young strategy and there's a good chance "exercise" will be the answer. And with good reason. Exercise, whether a gentle walk around the block or a full-tilt weight lifting session, strengthens the heart, lowers the body's resting heart rate, builds muscles, boosts circulation to the body and the brain, revs up the metabolism and burns calories. All of which can keep a person look and feel his or her best. To be effective, exercise must be performed several times a week. Aim for at least three sessions. However, there's more than one kind of exercise. For optimum health, try a combination of aerobic exercise and strength training. And don't forget to stretch before and after each workout!

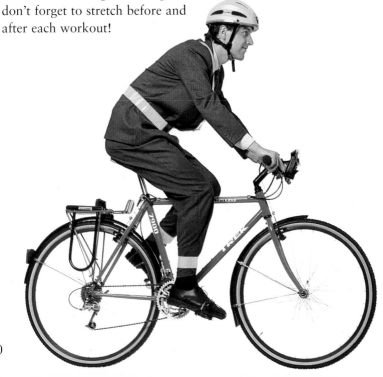

STRETCHING

❏ **What It Is:** Any movement that stretches muscles. Examples include bending at the waist and touching the toes, sitting with legs outstretched in front of you, and rolling your neck. Stretch for eight to twelve minutes before every workout and again after you exercise.

❏ **Why It's Important:** Muscles act like springs. If a muscle is short and tight, it loses the ability to absorb shock. The less shock a muscle can absorb, the more strain there is on the joints. Thus, stretching maintains flexibility, which in turn prevents injuries. Because we often lose our regular range of motion with age, stretching is especially important for older adults to prevent sprains, strains and falls.

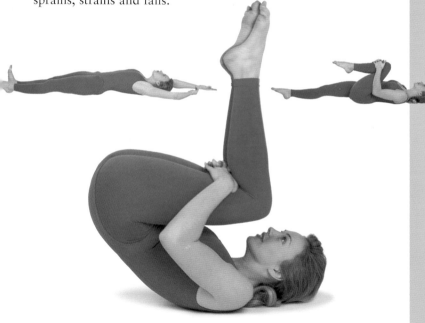

GET MOVING

AEROBICS

❐ **What It Is:** Any activity that uses large muscle groups, is maintained continuously for 15 minutes or more and is rhythmic in nature. Examples include aerobic dance, jogging, skating and walking. Ideally, you should aim for three to six aerobic workouts per week.

❐ **Why It's Important:** Aerobic exercise trains the heart, lungs and cardiovascular system to process and deliver oxygen more quickly and efficiently to every part of the body. As the heart muscle becomes stronger and more efficient, a larger amount of blood can be pumped with each stroke. Fewer strokes are then required to rapidly transport oxygen to all parts of the body.

STRENGTH TRAINING

❏ **What It Is:** Any activity that improves the condition of your muscles by making repeated movements against a force. Examples include lifting large or small weights, sit-ups, stair-stepping, and isometrics.

❏ **Why It's Important:** Strength training makes it easier to move heavy loads, whether they require carrying, pushing, pulling or lifting, as well as to
participate in sports that require strength. The exercises are of various kinds. Some require changing the length of the muscle while maintaining the level of tension,
others involve using special equipment to vary the tension in the muscles, and some entail contracting a muscle while maintaining its length.

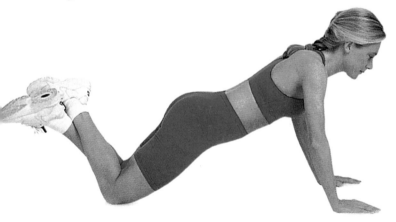

EATING SMART

A balanced diet is the foundation of good health. For proof, just read the numerous medical studies that link healthy eating with disease prevention and disease reversal. These same studies connect high fat intake, high sodium consumption and diets with too much protein to numerous illnesses, including cancer, cardiovascular diseases, diverticular diseases, hypertension and heart disease. But what exactly is a balanced diet? Generally speaking, it is a diet comprised of carbohydrates, dietary fiber, fat, protein, water, 13 vitamins and 20 minerals. More specifically, it is a diet built around a wide variety of fruits, legumes, whole grains and vegetables. Alcohol, animal protein, high-fat foods, high-sodium foods, highly-sugared foods, sodas and processed foods are consumed sparingly, if at all.

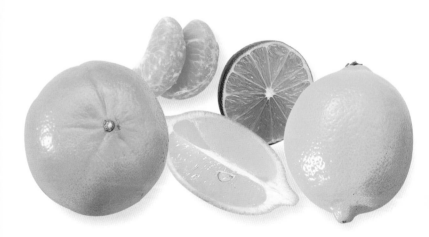

OMNIVOROUS

❒ **On The Menu:** Plant-based foods, dairy products, eggs, fish, seafood, red meats, organ meats, poultry.

❒ **Foods That Are Avoided:** None. Everything is fair game.

❒ **How Healthy Is It?** It depends. Someone who eats eggs, poultry or meat every day, chooses refined snacks over whole foods and gets only one or two daily servings of fruits and vegetables will not be as healthy as an omnivore who limits meat (the general dietary term for any "flesh foods," including poultry and fish) to two or three times a week, chooses water over soft drinks, and gets the recommended five or more daily servings of fruits and vegetables. Complaints about traditional omnivorous diets revolve around the diet's high level of cholesterol and saturated fat (found in animal-based foods), which increases one's risk of cancer, diabetes, heart disease and obesity.

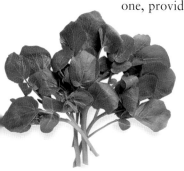

However, an omnivorous diet can be a healthy one, provided thoughtful choices are made. To keep cholesterol and saturated fat to a minimum and nutrients to a maximum, eat five or more daily servings of fruits and vegetables, choose whole grains over refined grains, enjoy daily legume or soyfood protein sources, and limit the use of animal foods.

EATING SMART

PISCATORIAL

❐ **On The Menu:** Plant-based foods, dairy products, eggs, fish, seafood.

❐ **Foods That Are Avoided:** Red meats, organ meats, poultry.

❐ **How Healthy Is It?** Like an omnivorous diet, a piscatorial diet is as healthy as a person makes it. Individuals who eat high-fat and highly processed foods fail to get the recommended daily number of vegetables and fruits, and eschew whole grains for processed grains will not enjoy optimum health. That said, individuals who are conscientious about eating a balanced, varied diet, and who limit fish and seafood intake to two or three times per week, can expect a lower risk of heart disease. Oily fish, eaten in moderation, has been found to help lower blood cholesterol, especially since many oily fish contain omega-3 fatty acids. Be aware, however, that oily saltwater fish, such as shark, swordfish and tuna, have been found to carry mercury in their tissues; many health authorities recommend eating these varieties no more than once or twice a week. Also, due to overfishing, many fish species are now threatened, including bluefin tuna, Pacific perch, Chilean sea bass, Chinook salmon, and swordfish. For additional information on endangered fish, visit the University of Michigan's Endangered Species Update at www.umich.edu/~esuupdate, or the Fish and Wildlife Information Exchange at http://fwie.fe.vt.edu.

MACROBIOTIC

❐ **On The Menu:** Plant-based foods, fish, very limited amounts of salt.

❐ **Foods That Are Avoided:** Dairy products, eggs, foods with artificial ingredients, hot spices, mass-produced foods, organ meats, peppers, potatoes, poultry, red meats, shellfish, warm drinks, refined foods.

❐ **How Healthy Is It?** Macrobiotics is based on a system created inn the early 1900s by Japanese philosopher George Ohsawa. The diet consists of 50 percent whole grains, 20 to 30 percent vegetables, and 5 to 10 percent beans, sea vegetables and soy foods. The remainder of the diet is composed of white-meat fish, fruits and nuts. The diet's low amounts of saturated fat, absence of processed foods, and emphasis on high-fiber foods, such as whole grains and vegetables, may promote cardiovascular health. Because soy and sea vegetables contain cancer-fighting compounds, macrobiotics is often recommended to help treat cancer. However, critics worry that the diet's limited variety of food can leave followers lacking in certain vitamins and important cancer-fighting phytonutrients.

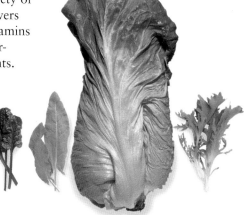

EATING SMART

VEGAN

❏ **On The Menu:** Plant-based foods.

❏ **Foods That Are Avoided:** Dairy, eggs, fish, seafood, red meats, organ meats, poultry. Also avoided are foods made by animals or processed with animal parts, such as gelatin, honey, marshmallows made with animal gelatin, white sugar processed with bone char.

❏ **How Healthy Is It?** A vegan (pronounced VEE-gun) diet can be extremely healthy. Like the vegetarian diet, a vegan diet has been shown by numerous studies to lower blood pressure and prevent heart disease. In addition, the high fiber intake cuts one's risk of diverticular disease and colon cancer. Yet, because vegans do not eat dairy products or eggs, they must be more conscientious than vegetarians about either eating plant foods with vitamin B_{12} and vitamin D, or taking supplements of these nutrients.

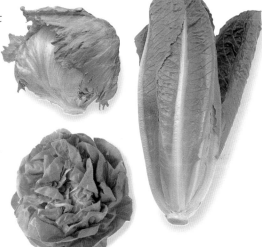

VEGETARIAN

❒ **On The Menu:** Plant-based foods, dairy, eggs.

❒ **Foods That Are Avoided:** Fish, gelatin, seafood, red meats, organ meats, poultry.

❒ **How Healthy Is It?** A vegetarian diet can be very healthy when done right. Fortunately, this isn't hard. Dietary science has debunked theories of "protein combining" popular in the 1960s and 1970s, leaving today's vegetarians to worry only about eating a wide variety of whole foods, including beans, fruits, grains, low-fat dairy products, nuts, soy foods, and vegetables. A varied daily diet insures enough protein, calcium and other nutrients for vegetarians of all ages, including children, pregnant individuals and the elderly. A well-chosen vegetarian eating plan has been shown by numerous studies to lower blood pressure, decrease one's risk of breast cancer and prevent heart disease. In addition, the diet's high fiber levels cuts the risk of diverticular disease and colon cancer.

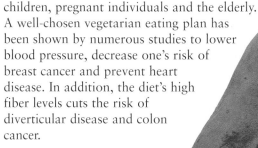

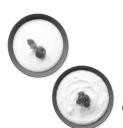

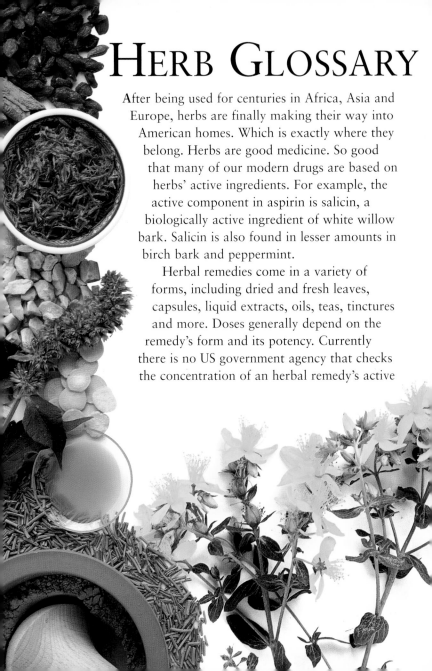

HERB GLOSSARY

After being used for centuries in Africa, Asia and Europe, herbs are finally making their way into American homes. Which is exactly where they belong. Herbs are good medicine. So good that many of our modern drugs are based on herbs' active ingredients. For example, the active component in aspirin is salicin, a biologically active ingredient of white willow bark. Salicin is also found in lesser amounts in birch bark and peppermint.

Herbal remedies come in a variety of forms, including dried and fresh leaves, capsules, liquid extracts, oils, teas, tinctures and more. Doses generally depend on the remedy's form and its potency. Currently there is no US government agency that checks the concentration of an herbal remedy's active

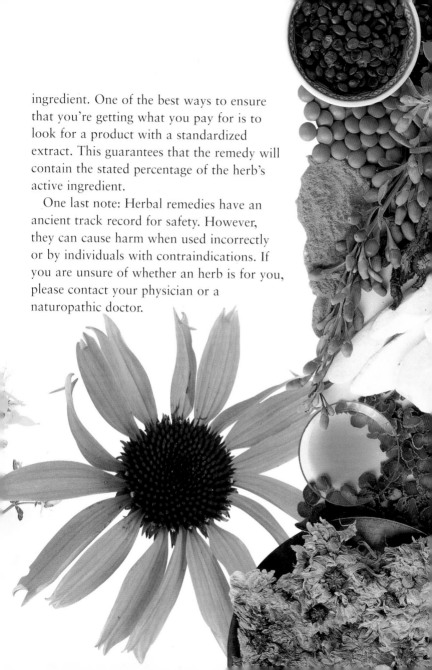

ingredient. One of the best ways to ensure that you're getting what you pay for is to look for a product with a standardized extract. This guarantees that the remedy will contain the stated percentage of the herb's active ingredient.

One last note: Herbal remedies have an ancient track record for safety. However, they can cause harm when used incorrectly or by individuals with contraindications. If you are unsure of whether an herb is for you, please contact your physician or a naturopathic doctor.

ALOE

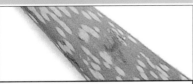

Properties: Analgesic, antibacterial, antifungal, anti-inflammatory, anti-itch, antiseptic, circulatory stimulant, digestive aid, immune-system stimulant, laxative.

Target Ailments: Acne, bruises, burns, constipation, cuts, insect bites, digestive disorders, rashes, ulcers, wounds.

Available Forms: Capsule, fresh leaves, gel, juice, liquid extract.

Possible Side Effects: When taken internally, aloe can cause severe cramping in some individuals.

Precautions: Pregnant women should not ingest aloe; It can stimulate uterine contractions.

CALENDULA

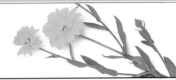

Properties: Antibacterial, anti-inflammatory, antiseptic, antispasmodic, promotes sweating, sedative.

Target Ailments: Burns, cuts, fungal infections, gallbladder conditions, hepatitis, indigestion, irregular menstruation, insect bites, menstrual cramps, mouth sores, skin rashes, ulcers, wounds.

Available Forms: Capsule, dried herb, fresh herb, liquid extract, lotion, oil, ointment, tincture.

Possible Side Effects: None expected.

Precautions: Calendula is related to ragweed. Individuals allergic to ragweed should consult a physician before using calendula.

ASTRAGALUS

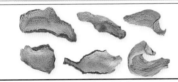

Properties: Antibacterial, anti-inflammatory, antioxidant, antiviral, diuretic, immune-system stimulant.

Target Ailments: Cancer, colds, appetite loss, diarrhea, fatigue, flu, heart conditions, HIV, viral infections.

Available Forms: Capsule, dried herb, fresh herb, liquid extract, tea, tincture.

Possible Side Effects: None expected.

Precautions: Astragalus should be used as a companion therapy to—not a replacement for—traditional cancer and HIV therapies.

CHAMOMILE

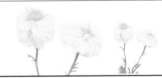

Properties: Antibacterial, anti-inflammatory, antiseptic, antispasmodic, carminative, digestive aid, fever reducer, sedative.

Target Ailments: Gingivitis, hemorrhoids, insomnia, indigestion, intestinal gas, menstrual cramps, nausea, nervousness, stomachaches, sunburns, tension, ulcers, varicose veins.

Available Forms: Capsule, dried herb, fresh herb, liquid extract, lotion, oil, tea, tincture.

Possible Side Effects: None expected.

Precautions: Because chamomile is related to ragweed, individuals with ragweed allergies should consult a physician before using chamomile.

DONG QUAI

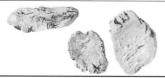

Properties: Antiallergenic, antispasmodic, diuretic, mild laxative, muscle relaxant, vasodilator.
Target Ailments: Abscesses, blurred vision, heart palpitations, irregular menstruation, light-headedness, menstrual pain, pallor, poor circulation.
Available Forms: Capsule, dried herb, liquid extract, tincture.
Possible Side Effects: Can cause photosensitivity in some individuals.
Precautions: Dong quai has abortive abilities; Do not take while pregnant.

FEVERFEW

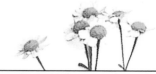

Properties: Anti-inflammatory, fever reducer.
Target Ailments: Arthritis, asthma, dermatitis, menstrual pain, migraines.
Available Forms: Capsule, dried herb, fresh herb, liquid extract, tincture.
Possible Side Effects: Some individuals experience "withdrawal" symptoms after taking feverfew, including fatigue and nervousness.
Precautions: Because it is related to ragweed, individuals with ragweed allergies should consult a physician before using feverfew.

ECHINACEA

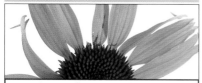

Properties: Antiallergenic, antibacterial, antiseptic, antimicrobial, antiviral, carminative, lymphatic tonic.
Target Ailments: Abscesses, acne, bladder infections, blood poisoning, burns, colds, eczema, food poisoning, flu, insect bites, kidney infections, mononucleosis, respiratory infections, sore throats.
Available Forms: Capsule, dried herb, liquid extract, tea, tincture.
Possible Side Effects: High doses can cause dizziness and nausea.
Precautions: Do not take echinacea for more than four weeks in a row.

GARLIC

Properties: Antibacterial, anticoagulant, antifungal, anti-inflammatory, antiviral, cholesterol reducer, digestive aid, immune-system stimulant, worm-fighting.
Target Ailments: Arteriosclerosis, arthritis, bladder infections, colds, digestive upset, flu, heart conditions, high blood pressure, high blood cholesterol, viral infections.
Available Forms: Capsule, fresh cloves, liquid extract, oil, tincture.
Possible Side Effects: Can cause upset stomach.
Precautions: While garlic is safe taken in culinary doses, individuals on anticoagulant medications should consult their doctors before supplementing their diet with garlic.

GINGER

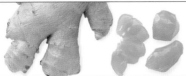

Properties: Antibacterial, anticoagulant, antinausea, antispasmodic, antiviral, carminative, digestive aid, expectorant, immune-system stimulant, muscle relaxant.
Target Ailments: Burns, colds, flu, high blood pressure, high cholesterol, liver conditions, intestinal gas, menstrual cramps, motion sickness, nausea, stomachaches.
Available Forms: Capsule, dried root, tea.
Possible Side Effects: Heartburn.
Precautions: While ginger is safe in culinary doses, individuals who suffer from a blood-clotting disorder or are on anticoagulant medication should consult a physician before supplementing their diet with the herb.

GINSENG

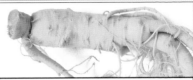

Properties: Antibacterial, antidepressant, immune-system stimulant, stimulant.
Target Ailments: Colds, depression, fatigue, flu, impaired immune system, respiratory conditions, stress.
Available Forms: Capsule, dried root, fresh root, liquid extract, tincture, tea.
Possible Side Effects: Large doses of ginseng can cause breast soreness, headaches or skin rashes in some individuals.
Precautions: Ginseng can aggravate existing heart palpitations or high blood pressure.

GINKGO BILOBA

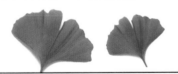

Properties: Antibacterial, anti-inflammatory, antioxidant, circulatory stimulant, vasodilator.
Target Ailments: Clotting disorders, dementia, depression, headaches, hearing loss, Raynaud's syndrome, tinnitus, vascular diseases, vertigo.
Available Forms: Capsule, dry herb, liquid extract, tincture, tea.
Possible Side Effects: Diarrhea, irritability, nausea, restlessness.
Precautions: Do not use ginkgo biloba if you have a blood-clotting disorder like hemophilia or are taking anticoagulant medications.

GOLDENSEAL

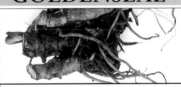

Properties: Antacid, antibacterial, antifungal, anti-inflammatory, antiseptic, astringent, digestive aid, stimulant.
Target Ailments: Canker sores, contact dermatitis, diarrhea, eczema, food poisoning.
Available Forms: Capsule, dry herb, liquid extract, tea, tincture.
Possible Side Effects: In high doses, goldenseal can cause diarrhea and nausea and can irritate the skin, mouth and throat.
Precautions: Because of its high cost, many manufacturers adulterate preparations with less costly herbs, such as barberry, yellow dock or bloodroot, some of which can cause unwanted reactions when taken in high doses.

KAVA

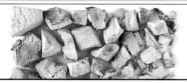

Properties: Antidepressant, antispasmodic, aphrodisiac, diuretic, muscle relaxant, sedative.
Target Ailments: Anxiety, colds, depression, menstrual conditions, muscle cramps, respiratory tract conditions, stress.
Available Forms: Capsule, dried herb, liquid extract, tea, tincture.
Possible Side Effects: Allergic skin reactions, muscle weakness, red eyes, sleepiness.
Precautions: In high doses, kava can impair motor reflexes and cause breathing problems.

MILK THISTLE

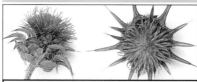

Properties: Anti-inflammatory, antioxidant, digestive aid, immune-system stimulant.
Target Ailments: inflammation of the gallbladder duct, hepatitis, liver conditions, poisoning from ingestion of the death cup mushroom, psoriasis.
Available Forms: Capsule, dried herb, fresh herb, powder, tea, tincture.
Possible Side Effects: Milk thistle can cause mild diarrhea when taken in large doses.
Precautions: If you think you have a liver disorder, seek medical advice before taking this herb.

LAVENDER

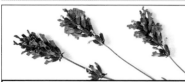

Properties: Antibacterial, antidepressant, antiseptic, antispasmodic, carminative, circulatory stimulant, digestive aid, diuretic, sedative.
Target Ailments: Anxiety, depression, headache, insomnia, intestinal gas, nausea, tension.
Available Forms: Capsule, dried herb, fresh herb, oil, tincture.
Possible Side Effects: Lavender products can cause skin irritation in sensitive individuals.
Precautions: Lavender oil is poisonous when ingested internally.

PARSLEY

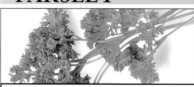

Properties: Antiseptic, antispasmodic, digestive aid, diuretic, laxative, muscle relaxant.
Target Ailments: Colds, congestion, fever, flu, indigestion, irregular menstruation, premenstrual syndrome, stimulating the production of breast milk, stomachaches.
Available Forms: Capsule, dried herb, fresh herb, liquid extract, oil, tea, tincture.
Possible Side Effects: Can cause photosensitivity in some individuals.
Precautions: Parsley should not be ingested in large amounts or used externally during pregnancy; it contains compounds that may stimulate uterine muscles and possibly cause miscarriage.

PEPPERMINT

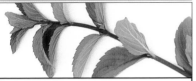

Properties: Antacid, antibacterial, antidepressant, antispasmodic, carminatve, expectorant, muscle relaxant, promotes sweating.
Target Ailments: Anxiety, colds, fever, flu, insomnia, intestinal gas, itching, migraines, morning sickness, motion sickness, nausea.
Available Forms: Capsule, dried herb, fresh herb, lozenge, oil, ointment, tea, tincture.
Possible Side Effects: When applied externally, peppermint products can cause skin reactions in sensitive individuals.
Precautions: If you have a hiatal hernia, talk to your doctor before using peppermint products externally or internally; the oil in the plant can exacerbate symptoms.

SAGE

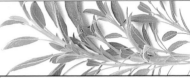

Properties: Antiseptic, anti-inflammatory, antioxidant, antispasmodic, astringent, bile stimulant, carminative, reduces perspiration.
Target Ailments: Excess intestinal gas, insect bites, menopausal night sweats, poor circulation, reduces milk flow at weaning, sore throat, stomachaches, mouth ulcers.
Available Forms: Capsule, dried herb, fresh herb, liquid extract, oil, tincture.
Possible Side Effects: Sage tea may cause inflammation of the lips and/or tongue in some individuals.
Precautions: Do not ingest pure sage oil; it is toxic when taken internally.

ROSEMARY

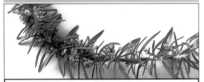

Properties: Antibacterial, antidepressant, anti-inflammatory, antiseptic, carminative, circultory stimulant.
Target Ailments: Bad breath, dandruff, depression, eczema, headaches, indigestion, joint inflammation, mouth and throat infections, muscle pain, psoriasis, rheumatoid arthritis.
Available Forms: Dried herb, fresh herb, ingestible rosemary-flavored oil, oil, ointment, tea, tincture.
Possible Side Effects: Rosemary oil can cause skin inflammation and/or dermatitis.
Precautions: Do not mistake regular rosemary oil for ingestible rosemary-flavored oil.

SAW PALMETTO

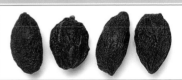

Properties: Antiallergenic, anti-inflammatory, diuretic, immune-boosting.
Target Ailments: Asthma, benign prostatic hyperplasia, bronchitis, colds, cystitis, impotence, male infertility, nasal congestion, sinus conditions, sore throats.
Available Forms: Capsule, dried herb, fresh herb, liquid extract, oil, tea, tincture.
Possible Side Effects: Can cause diarrhea if taken in large doses.
Precautions: Due to its hormonal actions, saw palmetto may interact negatively with prostate medicines or hormonal treatments such as estrogen replacement therapy, possibly canceling out their effectiveness.

ST. JOHN'S WORT

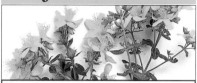

Properties: Analgesic, antibacterial, anti-depressant, anti-inflammatory, antiviral, astringent.

Target Ailments: Attention deficit disorder, anxiety, bacterial infections, burns, carpal tunnel syndrome, depression, HIV, menopause.

Available Forms: Capsule, dried herb, liquid extract, oil, ointment, tea, tincture.

Possible Side Effects: Gastrointestinal upset, headaches, photosensitivity, stiff neck.

Precautions: Avoid foods containing the amino acid tyramine when taking St. John's wort; the interaction of the two can cause an increase in blood pressure. Foods with tyramine include beer, coffee, wine, chocolate and fava beans.

WILD YAM

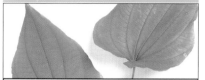

Properties: Analgesic, anti-inflammatory, antispasmodic, expectorant, muscle relaxant, promotes sweating.

Target Ailments: Menopause, menstrual cramps, morning sickness, nausea, rheumatoid arthritis, urinary tract infections.

Available Forms: Capsule, cream, dried root, liquid extract, oil, powder, tincture.

Possible Side Effects: Can cause vomiting in large doses.

Precautions: Individuals who are suffering from a hormone-sensitive cancer, such as breast or uterine cancer, should avoid wild yam. Some experts believe that the herb can encourage the growth of cancer cells.

VALERIAN

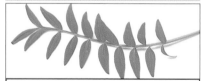

Properties: Analgesic, antibacterial, antispasmodic, carminative, reduces blood pressure, sedative, tranquilizer.

Target Ailments: Brachial spasm, high blood pressure, insomnia, palpitations, menstrual pain, migraines, muscle cramps, nervousness, tension headaches, wounds.

Available Forms: Capsules, dried herb, liquid extract, oil, teas, tincture.

Possible Side Effects: Headaches with prolonged use.

Precautions: Do not take with other sedatives, including alcohol. Do not drive or operate machinery after taking valerian.

YARROW

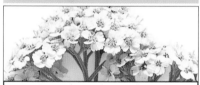

Properties: Antibacterial, anti-inflammatory, antispasmodic, blood coagulator, bile stimulating, immune-system stimulant, promotes sweating, sedative.

Target Ailments: Anxiety, colds and flu, cystitis, digestive disorders, menstrual cramps, minor wounds, nosebleeds, poor circulation, skin rashes.

Available Forms: Dried herb, capsule, liquid extract, oil, tea, tincture.

Possible Side Effects: Diarrhea, skin rash.

Precautions: Yarrow is related to ragweed and can cause an allergic reaction in individuals with ragweed allergies. Do not take if pregnant; it can induce miscarriage.

HERBAL TERMS

You're thumbing through the latest herbal therapy book when you run smack into the word "emmenagogue." Or perhaps you get tangled on "oxytocic." For anyone who's ever been stopped by an unfamiliar alternative medical term, we offer the following list:

Adaptogenic: Increases resistance and resilience to stress. Supports adrenal gland functioning.

Alterative: Blood purifier that improves the condition of the blood, improves digestion, and increases the appetite. Used to treat conditions arising from or causing toxicity.

Analgesic: Herb that relieves pain either by relaxing muscles or reducing pain signals to the brain.

Anthelmintic: Destroys or expels intestinal worms.

Antacid: Neutralizes excess stomach and intestinal acids.

Antiallergenic: Inactivates allergenic substances in the body.

Antibacterial/Antibiotic: Helps the body fight off harmful bacteria.

Antidepressant: Helps maintain emotional stability.

Anticatarrhal: Eliminates or counteracts the formation of mucus.

Anticoagulant: Thins blood and helps prevent blood clots.

Antifungal: Kills infection-causing fungi.

Anti-inflammatory: Reduces swelling of the tissues.

Anti-itch: Deadens itching sensations.

Antimicrobial: Kills a wide range of harmful bacteria, fungi, and viruses.

Antioxidant: Fights harmful oxidation.

Antipyretic/Fever Reducer: Reduces or prevents fever.

Antiseptic: External application prevents bacterial growth on skin.

Antispasmodic: Prevents or relaxes muscle tension.

Antiviral: Helps the body fight invading viruses.

Astringent: Has a constricting or binding effect. Commonly used to treat hemorrhages, secretions and diarrhea.

Blood Coagulant: Thickens blood and aids in clotting.

Carminative: Relieves gas.

Cholagogue: Encourages the flow of bile into the small intestine.

Circulatory Stimulant: Promotes even and efficient blood circulation.

Demulcent: Soothing substance, usually mucilage, taken internally to protect injured or inflamed tissues.

Diaphoretic: Induces sweating.

Diuretic: Increases urine flow.

Emetic: Induces vomiting.

Emmenagogue: Promotes menstruation.

Emollient: Softens, soothes and protects skin.

Expectorant: Assists in expelling mucus from the lungs and throat.

Galactogogue: Increases the secretion of breast milk.

Hemostatic: Stops hemorrhaging and encourages blood coagulation.

Hepatic: Tones and strengthens the liver.

Hypotensive: Lowers abnormally elevated blood pressure.

Immune-System Stimulant: Strengthens immune system so the body can fight off invading organisms.

Laxative: Promotes bowel movements.

Lithotriptic: Helps dissolve urinary and biliary stones.

Muscle Relaxant: Loosens tight muscles and reduces muscle cramping.

Nervine: Calms tension.

Oxytocic: Stimulates uterine contractions.

Rubefacient: Increases blood flow at the surface of the skin.

Sedative: Quiets the nervous system.

Sialagogue/Digestive Aid: Promotes the flow of saliva.

Stimulant: Increases the body's energy.

Tonic: Promotes the functions of body systems.

Vasoconstrictor: Constricts blood vessels, limiting the amount of blood flowing to a particular area.

Vasodilator: Dilates blood vessels, helping to promote blood flow.

Vulnerary: Encourages wound healing by promoting cell growth and repair.

HERBAL ORGANIZATIONS

Where to go for more information:

American Botanical Council
P.O. Box 201660
Austin, TX 78720
512-331-8868
www.herbalgram.org

The American Herbalist Guild
P.O. Box 746555
Arvada, CO 80006
303-423-8800

American Herbalists Guild
Box 1683
Soquel, CA 95073
408-464-2441

Herb Research Foundation
1007 Pearl Street, Suite 200
Boulder, CO 80302
303-449-2265
www.herbs.org

National Accupuncture and Oriental Medicine Alliance
14637 Starr Road SE
Olalla, WA 98359
206-851-6896

National Institutes of Health Office of Alternative Medicine
9000 Rockville Pike
Building 31, Room 5B-37
Mailstop 2182
Bethesda, MD 20892
301-402-2466

The Herb Society of America
9019 Kirtland-Chardon Road
Kirtland, OH 44094
216-256-0514

American College of Sports Medicine
P.O. Box 1440
Indianapolis, IN 46206
317-637-9200

American Heart Association
7272 Greenville Avenue
Dallas, TX 75231
214-373-6300

National Health Information Center
P.O. Box 1133
Washington, DC 20013
800-336-4797

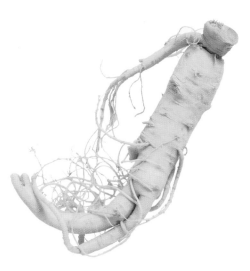

GROWING HERBS

Interested in cultivating herbs yourself?
These sources can supply roots, plants, and/or seeds.

Catoctin Mountain Botanicals
P.O. Box 454
Jefferson, MD 21755
301-473-4351

Companion Plants
7247 N. Coolville Ridge Rd.
Athens, OH 45701
614-593-3092
E-mail: complants@frognet.net

Dry Fork Herb Gardens
R.R.#1 Box 21
Rockport, IL
217-437-5281

Ecofriendly Farms
15488 Barn Rock Rd.
Mendota, VA 24270
540-466-8689

Goodwin Creek Gardens
P.O. Box 83
Williams, OR 97544
541-846-7357

Herbal Exchange
P.O. Box 429
9160 Lentz Rd.
Frazeysburg, OH 43822
614-828-9968

Horizon Herbs
P.O. Box 69
Williams, OR 97544
541-846-6233
www.chatlink.com/~herbseed
E-mail: herbseed@chatlink.com

Johnny's Seeds
Rt. 1 Box 2580
Foss Hill Rd.
Albion, ME 04910
207-437-9294
www.johnnyseeds.com

Mountain Traditions
H.C. 68, Box 193
Big Creek, KY 40914
606-598-6904

Nature's Cathedral
Rt. 1 Box 120
Blairstown, IA 52209
319-454-6959

Prairie Moon Nursery
Rt. 3, Box 163
Winona, MN 55987
507-452-1362

Wilcox Natural Products
P.O. Box 391
755 George Wilson Rd.
Boone, NC 28607
828-264-3615
www.goldenseal.com

Wild Wonderful Farm, Inc.
P.O. Box 256
Franklin, WV 26268
212-736-1467

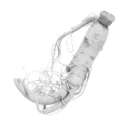

INDEX